Day by day, my body is transforming into the vision
I have for it.

Today I am healthy, strong, and disease-free!

I pay attention to the needs of my body. I feed it, exercise it, and love it!

I love my body and today I treat it with the respect it deserves.

I struggle, but I grow. I fall, but I get up.

I always train with intensity

Today I cease my focus on the weight I have to lose and focus completely on the me I am creating!

Today nothing, and I mean nothing, stands between me and my goal weight. I am there before I know it!

My body maintains its ideal weight and health

My body is the very picture of health and vitality!

I am dedicated to improving my fitness

Today I choose health and wellness over illness in my life.

I radiate good health.

Today I am making peace with food.

Who I am transcends a number on a scale! Today I focus on my health not my weight!

I am healthy and happy.

I appreciate and love my body

I love and accept myself at my current weight, even as I march pound by pound to my goal weight!

I am fit, healthy and attractive.

Breathing in, I feel healthy. Breathing out, I AM healthy.

I appreciate and love my body

My lungs breathe clear and strong!

Today I am transforming my body into
calorie-burning machine.

I love feeling fit and strong.

I have all the energy I need to accomplish my goals.

Today I exercise for my goal weight!

Today I see myself at my goal weight.

I AM healthy in mind, body, and spirit!

Today I release the need to weigh one pound more than I want to!

My life is what I make of it and today I choose to
make it healthy place to be.

I choose to be at a healthy weight

Today and every day, I cleanse my being with the life force of my breath.

Today I am making the choices and the changes to
have the body I want!

My heart beats strong and healthy!

I cannot lose 100 pounds this week, but I CAN lose three pounds and I AM!

Day by day, I am losing the weight and the people around me are taking notice.

My body is a marvelous machine that supports and meets my every need!

Even at the height of my pain, I experience moments of release, contentment, and joy.

I love and care for my body and it cares for me.

My sleep is relaxed and refreshing.

I am focused and motivated

I am full of energy

I am focused on achieving a high level of fitness

Today I am shedding the pounds as I shred my self doubt.

My pain is limited to my body.

I eat healthy and nutritious foods

Step by step and rep by rep, I am losing pounds and inches today!

Food nourishes my body, but I nourish my soul.

Every day, in every way, I am becoming better and better.

Today I eat for my goal weight!

Today I am blessed by the beautiful and delicious food that brings me to full health!

Today I experience vibrant health and profound well-being!

I am slender, strong, and perfectly conditioned.

Even amid adversity, I keep moving towards my goal weight.

Today I am seeing the new, slimmer me in the mirror and I love that!

I eat only to fuel my body when needed

I am filled with energy for all the daily activities in my life.

Today and every day, I feel the momentum building in my life for a healthy, fit lifestyle.

The older I get the healthier I become

I am healthy, happy and radiant.

I am beautiful, I am fit, I am healthy

I have abundant energy, vitality and well-being.

Today and every day, I express my gratitude for my good health.

I am extremely fit

My workout is something I look forward to

My weight is meaningless in the big picture.

It is easy for me to eat well and exercise regularly

Today I am shedding pounds as i shred my self-doubt!

My weight loss is within me. My diet is only a tool to get me to my goal.

My stamina is high

and more so every day!

My contributions to life measure my self-worth not the scale!

I am fit! I am healthy! I am strong!

As my reasons for holding on to my excess weight melt away, so does the weight.

Today I push my limits in the gym so that tomorrow
I can push the limits in my life!

The longer I exercise the stronger I get and the stronger I get the longer I exercise!

My mind is at peace.

Pound by pound, inch by inch, choice by choice I
am becoming healthy and fit!

As my self-confidence rises, the number on the
scale drops!

My body is healed, restored and filled with energy.

Step by step and rep by rep, I am creating my ideal body!

I have a strong desire to be healthy and strong

My immune system is healthy, strong, and protecting me right now!

When I feel good, I exercise. When I exercise, I feel good.

Day by day, I am transforming my body into a high performance machine!

Today my portion size is shrinking and so is my waistline.

My body is a well-oiled machine ready to meet my every need!

I live a healthy lifestyle

I beyond the need for food to fill me up. My life is full of people and activities that do it.

Day in and day out, I develop the habits of health!

A fit, healthy person lives within me. Today that person emerges.

I may have to live with pain, but I absolutely refuse
to be defined by it!

I am constantly connected to something far greater than my body.

My fitness routine is interesting and varied

As I commit to my exercise program, I transform my body!

Today I weigh less than yesterday and tomorrow I weigh even less!

Happiness is an attitude not a number on a scale! I refuse to be defined by my weight!

I deserve a healthy, fit body and today I claim it!

I am strong, vibrant, and healthy!

I am calm and at peace

Today I AM my goal weight!

9 781730 975936